THE SIX RULES OF FITNESS FOR LIFE

Your Simple Action Plan for Living Your Best Life After 40

by

BECKY WILLIAMSON, M.S.

CONTENTS

Dedication

I dedicate this book to all the folks out there over 40 who are taking charge of their bodies and putting effort into staying healthy and feeling their best while they travel through "mid-life."

We're changing what "older" looks and feels like, my friends!

Acknowledgments

First and foremost, I'd like to thank my husband, Matt Repanich, for being my biggest cheerleader and for always believing in me—even when I didn't believe in myself. I love you so much and truly appreciate your unconditional support of my business activities through the years.

Thank you to Pat Rigsby for suggesting I write this book, for all your years of coaching and for your patience.

I'd also like to thank all my clients—past and present. It is because of you that I have been able to do what I love for a living. It is helping you feel better and improving your health that brings me joy. Thank you for bringing joy to my life.

Preface

Hello and thank you so much for picking up this book! I hope you find it educational and informative and that it provides just the motivation you need to take the next step toward maintaining or improving your fitness.

I decided to write this book because I wanted to share what I believe are the best practices with regard to maintaining a healthy lifestyle after the age of 40. There is so much conflicting information out there with relative to the best exercise plan or the best eating plan. It can get really confusing. The confused mind often takes no action at all (ever heard of the phrase "paralysis by analysis?"). My goal for you with this book is to help dispel some myths, simplify some concepts and give you suggestions on actions you can take to live your best life after 40.

I don't believe that there is a "one size fits all" plan for everyone. We're all individuals. What works for one person might not work for the next person. But of this I am sure: You can do something today to be better tomorrow. You absolutely, positively can improve your current situation. All of us can eat better, exercise smarter and decrease our risk for disease starting today. How we put it all together to make it work with our goals and our lifestyle is where the differences come into play.

I have worked with a wide range of ages and abilities over the last 30 years, but now I specialize in training the over-40 population. Although I accept clients younger than 40, I really love working with the over-40 crowd. The time in life when men and women approach and enter their 40's is often a time they tell me they really feel their body is different and that it's not responding the way it has in the past with regard to exercise and nutrition. I feel a special "kinship" with those of you who are experiencing changes in how your body feels, looks and moves because...I've been there. With quite a few years under my belt helping busy people stay in shape, I've also learned a thing or two about what works best concerning exercise and nutrition after 40.

A lot of prospective clients come to me tired, feeling flabby and out of shape. They are often in some sort of pain and are frustrated that their exercise efforts haven't resulted in any measurable results. They've often attended large group exercise classes where they weren't really noticed and they ended up getting hurt. So they now believe exercise just doesn't work for them. These people often tell me they feel their age creeping up on them at a much faster pace in recent years. Some even feel they're resigned to "getting old" because they can't quite figure out how to go about staying fit. If you've felt this way, please keep reading, as I have some tricks up my sleeve to help you re-claim your feelings of youth and vitality.

Because you picked up this book, I'm guessing that feeling good and moving well are important to you. Throughout the chapters in this book, I will walk you through some basic ideas that you can apply to your daily life. Most people come to me for a plan and some guidance. That is what I will provide for you here.

You see, the basics of getting fit and staying fit are, well, kind of basic. We just need to be able to cut through the conflicting information to find out what works best for you.

I will guide you toward looking and feeling your best with some really simple, straightforward tips. As we age, it can be hard to figure out how our workout and nutrition strategies need to change as our body and our lifestyle changes throughout the years. I'm guessing there are days when you are reminded that you're not 25 anymore. As I write this, I've passed my 58th birthday, so I truly do understand your experiences with changes in hormones, metabolism and joints at this point in your life. In general, I enjoy a healthy, active life and consider myself pretty fit. But it's just different type of fit than when I was 25, or even when I was 35. I'm guessing you might be nodding your head right now. A 40 or 50-year old body can still be (and should be) healthy and fit—we just may need to do things just a little differently now.

Introduction

I believe that everyone needs a coach at various times in their life. Athletes use coaches. CEO's use coaches. I use a coach to help me build my business. Coaches help their clients achieve more and do more than they can on their own. My hope is that I'll be able to be your coach here (at least for the length of this book) and help you sift through the myths, truths and half-truths that are out there with regard to the best way to exercise and eat in your 40's, 50's and beyond.

I've divided this book into 6 sections or "Rules" which I believe individuals over 40 need to embrace and implement into their lifestyle in order to live the best, healthiest, most active life possible. Could I have added more than 6 Rules? Absolutely! But I decided to narrow it down and give you the "Cliff's Notes" version on what I think are the most important and profound concepts for being fit after 40.

I could probably write a whole book on each one of the Rules I've listed, but I've given you what I think are the best nuggets of wisdom to help you navigate your health and fitness over the age of 40. After I present to you each of my Rules, I end the chapter with a suggested action plan for you. If you're reading a Rule and it really resonates with you and you feel you really need to work on that area—you'll find some suggested steps at the end of each chapter to help you get focused and take action.

I believe the information in this book can help you change the course of your life.

However, information without action will get you nowhere.

Please commit to taking action on at least ONE of the Rules you read. I promise it will help improve some facet of your well-being.

One of the mottos of my company, lifeSport Fitness, is "Life's More Fun When You're Fit." Living life in a body that is sick, tired, and out of shape just doesn't sound like much fun, does it? The wonderful thing is that it is within your power to "live young" and make improvements in your current state of health if you're not in ideal health right now. If you're healthy and fit, the guidelines in this book will support you in your quest to stay that way and will give you some new ideas to try as well. I'm excited to walk you through this journey, so let's get started.

Before we dive in, one quick note: I want take a moment to explain a term you'll see throughout this book. I use the term "fat loss" throughout this book. When clients come to me for coaching, they often state they want to "lose weight." I understand what they are looking for in terms of results. They really are asking for fat loss. I take time to explain how scale weight (the weight they are telling me they wish to lose) does not tell the whole story.

I'd like to explain it here to you so that we're on the same page.

Although there is nothing wrong with weighing yourself on a bathroom scale, that number on the scale doesn't tell us how much of your weight is fat and how much of your weight is water, muscles, bones, organs, etc. If we only look at dropping scale weight, we could be doing ourselves a disservice. "Dieting" profusely (especially if you are not doing any sort of strength training) can really change the number on your bathroom scale. However, that scale doesn't tell you if you've lost muscle or bone along the way. Losing too much "weight" from dieting when you're over 40 can be a real problem. You might diet away muscle (and potentially bone). You need that muscle. You need strong bones. Muscle burns calories all day long and muscle is what will keep you independent as you age.

Therefore, when clients tell me they want to lose weight what I hear is "fat loss" and I set out to design a program that will help them slim down, but still maintain their lean mass (bones and muscle). When you see the term "fat loss" in this book, I'm referring to the same thing my clients who want to lose weight are referring to. I use the term "fat loss" because it's truly what we're after.

WHAT IS NORMAL AGING, ANYWAY?

A common thought amongst individuals over 40 is that we just get slower, fatter and more out of shape as we age. You've probably even heard reports that "your metabolism slows as you age" and "you'll lose muscle every decade of your life after the age of 40."

Are these reports true? Well, yes. But...maybe not.

You see, much of the early research done on "older" test subjects was done on sedentary individuals. It's now thought the age-related decline seen in older adults really isn't age-related at all. It's really more related to lack of activity and a sedentary lifestyle. Genetics, diet, smoking, alcohol use and, especially, lack of physical activity, may all contribute to this decline.

What would happen if we looked at physically active older adults in a study? A 2011 study of recreational cyclists aged 40-81, showed no significant decline in thigh musculature or thigh strength due to age. Aging is commonly associated with a loss of muscle mass and strength, resulting in falls, functional decline, and the subjective feeling of weakness. This study contradicts the common observation that muscle mass and strength decline as a function of aging alone. The study authors suggested that these declines may signal the effect of chronic disuse rather than muscle aging[1].

A 2010 study looked at the shin musculature in older (average age, 65 years) recreational runners and compared the muscle tissue to the shin muscles in younger (average age, 25 years) recreational runners[2]. The older runner's shin muscles had nearly the

[1] https://www.ncbi.nlm.nih.gov/pubmed/22030953
Phys Sportsmed. 2011 Sep;39(3):172-8. doi: 10.3810/psm.2011.09.1933.
Chronic exercise preserves lean muscle mass in master athletes.
[2] Med Sci Sports Exerc. 2010 Sep;42(9):1644-50. doi: 10.1249/MSS.0b013e3181d6f9e9.
Motor unit number estimates in masters runners: use it or lose it?
Power GA1, Dalton BH, Behm DG, Vandervoort AA, Doherty TJ, Rice CL.

same amount of motor units as the young runners. The more motor units in a muscle, the stronger it is – so the older runners were maintaining their leg strength and muscle health by running. These are just two studies, but I assure you we're seeing more and more studies on active older adults that show recreational activities are preserving muscle mass well into people's 6th and 7th decades. Wow! Powerful stuff.

I don't want to make this book a research review, but just wanted to make the point that the tapes we play in our mind and the discussions we have in our social circles about what "normal" aging is may be a bit flawed. I'd like to call them urban legends. Some of those concepts are from information gathered a long time ago. Some of it is from anecdotal evidence from watching our parents and grandparents. As I've shown you, we've got new data on a new generation of "older" people. These new data are proving that we might not be getting out of shape because we're older. We may be getting out of shape and feeling old because we're moving less and/or making poor food choices.

Look at some active older adults you know (maybe you can look in the mirror on this one), and I'd bet that those you are looking at are more youthful and active at their current age than their own grandparents were at the same age. I'd like to think that you and I and all the wonderful people over 40 that I currently train are re-defining what it looks and feels like to age into our 40's, 50's and beyond.

So, after our mini research review there, let's revisit those common concepts of "your metabolism slows as you age" and "you'll lose muscle every decade of your life after the age of 40" and consider this question: Is it possible that by maintaining an active lifestyle, using and challenging our muscles, eating whole, unprocessed foods and keeping our calorie intake in check that we might slow the aging process?

Yes!

I truly believe (and research studies support) the notion that staying active and maintaining your muscle mass will slow down the functional decline we may have seen in our grandparents when they were our age. Chronic disuse, poor lifestyle habits and poor nutrition, rather than the function of aging alone is probably why some of us get "old" too young.

So, here we are. The years have flown by and you find yourself now over the age of 40. Do you have to settle with feeling old? Do you have to settle for a metabolism that seems to be coming to a screeching halt? Are achy joints something you just have to deal with?

To these questions, I say an emphatic "No!" I believe it's within your power to feel great, move well, decrease pain and feel youthful for much longer than you might imagine simply by changing a few daily habits. If you've got a retirement "bucket list" to get through, the steps I lay out for you here will help you get through that bucket list a lot faster with increased energy, more strength, less pain and a whole lot more fun (life's more fun when you're fit, remember?).

My goal with this book is to guide you through the process of living your BEST life now. I want to show you how you can feel younger and more energetic.

To do this correctly and safely, though, I'd suggest you follow the rules outlined in this book.

The Rules

1. Find your "why"
2. Train for the goal
3. Mind your muscle
4. Recovery matters
5. Be flexible
6. You can't out-train a poor diet

1

Rule #1: Find Your Why

I think it's safe to assume that you have probably hopped on and fallen off the exercise/eat healthier wagon a few times in the last few decades, right? Don't feel bad. It happens to the best of us.

Why do we start an exercise routine or healthy eating plan only to stop it weeks or months later? Lots of reasons: Perceived lack of time, boredom, lack of results, injury...and the list goes on. Our logical mind tells us "this is good for you," but we still don't make the effort after a period of time.

It's natural for our motivation levels to ebb and flow at times. However, to be successful in adopting healthy habits and a fitness lifestyle, I encourage you to really dig deep and find your "why."

Why is improving your health and fitness important to you?

Why do you want to have more energy?

Or a smaller waistline?

Or less knee pain?

This is why I list "Find Your Why" as Rule #1. When the going gets tough as you work on new lifestyle habits (the other 5 Rules), your "why" will help you keep going and stay focused.

Your why has to be important to YOU. It can't be because someone else wants it for you. It does need to be something you want deeply at your core. It has to be truly important to you. Things that aren't truly important to you tend to take a back seat in your life after a while.

Now, you might think when I ask you "what are your fitness goals?" I'm asking you for your why. Nope. That's the "what." Examples of your "what" might be:

- to lose a few inches in your waistline
- to decrease your blood sugar
- to be able to touch your toes or bend your knees without pain

Once you've expressed your "what" as specifically as possible, then it's time to get to your why. My experience has shown that the first few answers I get when I ask a client for the "why" to their goals aren't really the real down-deep "why." We have to peel down a few layers first.

Let me illustrate how we can peel down to the real why with a series of questions and answers with a fictitious new client we'll call Bob.

Coach Becky: "So, Bob, what are your goals?"

Bob: "I want to decrease my belly size and lower my blood sugar level."

Coach Becky: "Okay, Bob, I can set up a program to help you do that. Why is a smaller belly and a lower blood sugar important to you?"

Bob: "Well, I don't want my belly to be this big and my doc says I should get my blood sugar under control."

Coach Becky: "Why does the size of your belly concern you, Bob? And why is your doctor telling you to decrease your blood sugar?"

Bob: "This gut makes me look like my Dad when he got older. Oh, and the doc says I'm borderline diabetic."

Coach Becky: "So, Bob, why does looking like your Dad concern you?"

Bob: "I don't want to end up like him."

Coach Becky: "Why not? What happened to him?"

Bob: "After retirement, my Dad stayed sedentary, continued to eat poorly and his diabetes got the best of him. He was old before his time and he died due to complications from his diabetes. I don't want to go down that path and I feel like I'm starting to."

Aha! So, once we "peel the onion" we learn it's not really *all* about aesthetics and a big belly is it? It's about wanting to avoid the fate of his Dad and the physical decline he saw happen with his father. *Now*, we're getting somewhere. This will be a much bigger motivator when the going gets tough rather than just the desire for a smaller waistline.

Coach Becky: "So Bob, it sounds like you're looking to decrease your belly size in order to decrease your risk for Type 2 Diabetes."

Bob: "Well, yeah, I guess that's what it comes down to."

Coach Becky: "Okay, Bob, talk to me about what your life might look like in 3-6 months if you start on a regular exercise program and healthy eating plan today."

What I'm doing here is having the client talk about the benefits they'll enjoy from sticking to their new program. It's really important that you list out what you'll enjoy/feel like/be able to do once your goals are met. You'll want to list these out so that you can refer to them when your motivation begins to lag.

Bob: "I'll feel better about myself, I'll fit into my pants and I'll decrease my risk for Type 2 diabetes and the health complications my Dad had."

Coach Becky: "Yes, Bob, you absolutely will and I'll be right here by your side helping you every step of the way. For a moment, let's look at the other side of the coin, though. What will happen if you don't make some exercise and lifestyle changes soon?"

It's always important to look at the flip side and visit the "what happens if I don't stick with this?" scenario when you're discovering your why.

Bob: "Oh, I don't even want to think about it. I'll stay overweight and out of shape, my blood sugar will continue to go up, and I'll end up in poor health like my Dad."

This illustration of a conversation I'd have to help someone discover their why is something you can do on your own, or with an interviewer to ask you the questions. The process will not only help you discover your why, but it will also help you outline the benefits you'll enjoy from beginning a regular exercise and healthy eating program. It will also force you to look at the other side of the situation if you aren't consistent with your program.

As a coach, my job is to help my clients stay as highly motivated as possible (highly motivated clients get the best results). I make it my job to understand each of my clients' motivational hot buttons and I try very hard to understand their why.

Most of us don't exercise for the sheer sake of spending our time exercising. Your workout (or your healthy eating plan) is a means to an end. But here's the thing—that "end" isn't your why. I want you to understand and embrace why you desire that end result.

If you're lifting weights, is it to be stronger? Okay, good. So you get stronger. Why is that important to you?

If you're doing yoga in an effort to be more flexible or to manage stress and you become more flexible and/or less stressed, why is that important?

You see, what I'm asking you here is to tell me why you want/need that end result of a workout program or a healthy eating regimen.

Peel the onion. Get to the real core.

Discovering your WHY and really focusing on it can help you maintain consistency and re-ignite your passion for exercise if you happen to lose momentum and get off track.

Allow me to give you a little coaching session here and help you find your "why" for exercising regularly and adopting a healthy eating program.

Here are a series of questions to help you discover your why. You may have several health or fitness goals you'd like to achieve, but for simplicity, choose one and run it through this series of questions.

1. List one health or fitness goal you'd like to achieve within the next 6 months.

2. Why is this goal important to you?

3. Why do you list the answer in question #2? Why is that significant?

4. Why does your answer to #3 matter to you?

5. What are the benefits you'll enjoy from achieving what you list in question #1?

6. What will happen/what will you feel like/what will your life be like if you stop working on this goal?

Your "why" should give you specific, meaningful motivation to continue with your exercise and healthy eating plan. Your "why" gives you motivation and a reason to keep going when you don't want to.

When you have a tough day or feel like you are losing momentum, return to this section to re-connect with why improving your health and fitness is important to you.

When you feel like quitting, think about why you started. "Because I'm supposed to" won't last very long. Whereas, "so I can get down on the ground to play w/my grandkids" or "so I don't get heart disease early like my mom did" may keep you a bit more focused and motivated.

I believe people over 40 need to let go of the "hurry up and lose weight/get fit in 6 weeks" mentality and ease into a regular program especially if you're starting from ground zero. We need to be patient with our bodies. Too much too soon usually isn't a good thing. It can derail you or lead to injury. Be realistic and consistent, and always keep your eye on your "why" to maintain focus.

I've created a "Find Your Why" worksheet for you. You'll find it in Appendix A. Use it to help you "peel the onion" and dig down to find what really, really matters to you and why getting healthier overall is important to you. Keep your completed checklist handy so that you can refer back to it if you get off track or find yourself losing motivation.

Your Action Plan

Dig in and work on the "Find Your Why" worksheet! Consider making a copy and putting it somewhere where you'll see it daily.

2

Rule #2: Train for the Goal

A lot of us over 40 have different goals than we did at 25. Back in our 20's we wanted to rock our skinny jeans or look good in swim trunks. Not that we don't want to look good now, but things like getting up off the floor without making too many groaning noises or chasing our grandkids at the park are higher priority on our list these days.

What are your most pressing issues now? Balance?
Mobility? Fat Loss? Strength? Endurance?
Decreasing disease risk? Whatever they might be,
your exercise (and nutrition program) should be
designed to help you improve those areas.

Exercise and healthy eating isn't really one size fits
all. We're all different. We have different needs,
different abilities and even different biochemistries
that will dictate how some foods or forms of exercise
affect us.

For that reason, it wouldn't be possible for me to
outline the ideal exercise program for you here since
I don't know your current physical abilities and your
goals. However, I'm going to give you some general
recommendations on what I think a person over 40
should strive for when creating a well-rounded
physical fitness program and healthy eating lifestyle
for themselves. In this chapter, we'll focus on
exercise. I've got a whole chapter on nutrition later
on.

First and foremost, I'd like for you to consider the
concept of "train for the goal." Although I believe

that, with few exceptions, all movement is good and we older folks should move a lot—some forms of exercise are better than others for certain goals. Case in point: If osteoporosis prevention is your goal, swimming or stationary cycling wouldn't be my first choices of exercise for you. They're both great for cardiorespiratory fitness and some muscle strength, but because they are not weight bearing exercise, these two modes shouldn't be your only forms of exercise if you're trying to maintain bone.

If you were my client and you told me you wanted to maintain your bone mass, we'd be doing weight-bearing cardiovascular conditioning as well as strength training (and ideally strength training while standing up – not sitting on machines). If your goal is fat loss, I would have you start building muscle by lifting weights. Yes, most people born in my era would think they should do lots of cardio to lose fat. Not so. Cardiovascular exercise has a place in a fat loss program, but adding muscle to your frame is king. The more muscle you have on your frame, the more calories you burn all day long.

Setting up the right exercise program that can actually lead to achieving your goals is really one of the most important rules at any age, but especially for those of us over 40.

There are a lot of canned training programs out there that give you the "Workout of the Day" when you walk in or the "Endurance" workout on Tuesday and the "Core" workout on Friday. But—what if that's not really what you need that day? What if you need more core strength and hip mobility to improve your golf swing, or you need lots of work on your hips and thighs to shore up an arthritic knee? In my experience, you need those foundational exercises as the base of your program and they should be done regularly – not just when they appear on the whiteboard at the gym.

As I've mentioned, I believe all forms of exercise are good, but when you're over 40, I'd like to see you really specialize and find just the right mix of strength, balance, mobility, agility and/or endurance that you need for whatever it is you want to accomplish. I'd like to see you find a workout plan that takes your current physical condition into consideration and has a progressive nature to it to safely and effectively advance you along the way.

It's hard to know how to start and what to do if you don't know what type of a program is best for your particular goals. I'd go a step further and tell you that sometimes what you want (for example, weight loss) is not the only thing you need. You might need some mobility work in order to be able to perform a strength training program safely and effectively. Bottom line: Sometimes you don't know what you don't know. This is where a qualified coach comes in.

Since I don't know you personally, I can't give you specific recommendations for exercise, but I'd like to give you some general recommendations that can help you begin the process of putting together a safe and effective exercise program to train for your goals.

Good choices if your goal is fat loss

Strength training
High Intensity Interval Training (more on this later in this chapter)

Longer, lower intensity cardiovascular exercise (this is listed third in importance for a reason)

Good choices if your goal is increased strength

Strength training
Cycling (this will improve lower body strength)
Treadmill running/walking on an incline (this will improve lower body strength a little)
Water aerobics
Group exercise classes with an emphasis on weight lifting (boot camps, circuit training, BodyPump™)

Good choices if your goal is cardiovascular endurance

Long distance brisk walking
Jogging
Swimming laps
Cycling
Group exercise classes (like Zumba, jazzercise, and traditional aerobic dance)

Good choices if your goal is stress management

Yoga
Pilates
Walking (especially with your dog)
Hiking
T'ai Chi

Good choices if your goal is improved balance

Yoga
Strength training
T'ai Chi
Some forms of martial arts
Specialty group exercise classes with balance as the focus

Many people that I train come to me to lose weight, and I go about creating a strength training and cardiovascular training program to get the results they're looking for. More often than not after I've done an assessment on them, though, I'll decide to sneak in a few exercises to work on things my clients don't even know they need.

Mobility and flexibility are two measures of fitness that stand out to me as areas of focus that should be a part of every person's physical fitness program if they're over 40. I see a lot of stiff joints and tight muscles in some of my clients who are busy Silicon Valley professionals. I think we have a term for it now and it's called it "Silicon Valley Syndrome." In Silicon Valley Syndrome, we see tight rear thigh muscles, tight chest muscles, stiff hips, and back and butt muscles that aren't as strong as they should be. This comes about from sitting a great deal of the work day and during the commute to/from work (and I bet people outside of Silicon Valley have this, too).

Bottom line: If your workout regimen creates the ability for you to move better overall and with greater ease, you will be more successful in your exercise pursuits as well as your recreational pursuits. Furthermore, when you move better, you'll likely move more often and get better results from your exercise efforts. An added bonus: You'll probably also be in less pain. Funny how that all comes together, isn't it?

To summarize, the main focus of your exercise program and where you spend the greatest amount of your time on exercise should be geared toward your main fitness/health goal, but consider throwing in some flexibility and mobility work as well. You may be moving better than your peers after a while.

If you're looking for an overall well-rounded exercise program as a person over the age of 40, I believe you should focus some of your exercise on improving these key components: Muscular strength, cardiovascular endurance, balance, mobility and flexibility.

What to do if your goal is weight loss

For many years, the common thought has been that if your goal is to lose weight, you need to eat a calorie-restricted low fat diet and do lots and lots of long cardio workouts. I'll address the nutrition component in a later chapter, but let's talk about those long cardio workouts now.

If you are a long distance runner, swimmer or cyclist, I'm not about to suggest that you stop. Keep doing what you're doing if it's serving your needs. However, if you believe you need to do hours of cardio to lose weight...read on.

You don't.

Most of the more recent studies on long cardio workouts (45+ minutes per session) are showing that they aren't that effective for weight loss. Don't get me wrong. Longer cardiovascular exercise sessions have great benefits for you. But, those longer cardio workouts may not be the best way or the only way to lose weight. They're definitely not the fastest way.

Research is showing that strength training and High Intensity Interval Training ("HIIT") produce better weight loss results (as does a change in your nutrition) than long duration, moderate to low intensity cardio workouts.

What is HIIT?

HIIT is an exercise technique in which you give all-out, near maximal effort with quick, intense bursts of exercise, followed by active recovery periods. This type of training is short in duration (usually 20 minutes or less and sometimes as little as 5 or 6 minutes). It's not easy to do, and it's something you need to work up to slowly if you're not used to it, but it can be very effective for weight loss and muscle preservation when combined with good nutrition.

Newer research findings suggest that these HIIT workouts of short bursts of high intensity exercise followed by active rest periods may offer better fat loss results. Athletes have done these types of interval workouts for years in an effort to improve aerobic capacity and speed, but now we're finding that these workouts may be good for the rest of us as well.

Studies show that doing these bursts of high intensity exercise improves the body's ability to burn fat in the hours after the exercise is over. In order to better understand these research findings, I contacted the lead researcher of one of the studies looking at HIIT exercise. Here is what he said in an email to me: "We have shown that interval training not only improves exercise performance and overall fitness, but it improves the potential of the muscle to burn fat during exercise. Now, this doesn't mean that interval training burns stored fat as we're doing the exercise, because we know that high intensity exercise requires a faster burning fuel like carbohydrate. But what it does tell us is that if you do interval training, it will improve your ability to burn fat during lower intensity exercise."

In addition to the knowledge that high intensity exercise makes us a better "fat burner" in our lower intensity exercise pursuits, we also know that very hard exercise seems to create an "after burn" effect wherein you burn more calories from stored fat in the hours after your HIIT workout. This effect has been seen repeatedly in dozens of studies and it now it has its own name: Excess post-exercise oxygen consumption. For the sake of this book, let's just stick with "after burn." It's a lot easier to say.

.

Here's how I see the value of HIIT workouts in relation to you and your weight loss goals: If you take a few of your longer, lower intensity cardio workouts and make them shorter, but more intense with high/low intensity segments, you'll burn more calories in those workouts than you would have at a lower intensity and you'll become a better fat burner during your moderate intensity workouts and if you work hard enough, you'll enjoy that "after burn" effect. What's more, you'll decrease your workout time by a large margin.

More results in less time. Sounds like good exercise math to me!

Oh, and there goes your "I don't have time to spend an hour at the gym" excuse.

How to do HIIT

There is no accepted formula for the ideal ratio between hard work and active rest periods. In fact, I believe the best thing to do is to mix it up. The body is very adaptable. If you keep changing your workout, your body can't adapt. This is actually a good thing. If it can't adapt because you keep changing things up, it has to work harder. Working harder burns more calories.

You don't need specialized equipment to do HIIT. In my personal training sessions, I offer an optional "finisher" at the end of the workout session where I cycle clients between work/recovery periods of 50 seconds:10 seconds, 40 seconds: 20 seconds, 35 seconds: 15 seconds or 20 seconds:10 seconds. Every week the timing is different, the number of work/recovery rounds the clients complete is different, and the exercises are different. They do fast squats and "skater" moves, they slam balls and heavy ropes, they hop or jump, or do any number of higher intensity callisthenic-type activities. This keeps my client's bodies working hard and never getting too efficient at performing one specific type of exercise.

In my own personal workouts, I've done running sprints on the straight part of the local high school track, and recovered around the curve in the track. No timer needed. The shape of the track and my running pace dictates my work/recovery times. You can do this on a hill as well. Walk or run up the hill, and then recover by returning to the bottom of the hill.

The possibilities are endless with regard to how you time your HIIT workout and the type of exercise you choose.

In Appendix B, I've written out a few simple HIIT ideas you can try at home or your gym.

A few important guidelines apply to High Intensity Interval Training:

- The high-intensity phase should be hard enough that you get out of breath.

- Recovery periods should not last long enough for your pulse to return to its resting level.

- Anyone with heart disease or high blood pressure should consult a physician before exercising, especially at very high intensities.

- If you're new to interval training, start with just one or two sessions a week, and fill in the week with moderate aerobic exercise. As you become more accustomed to interval work, you can add in another interval day.

Barring any health or musculoskeletal issues that would prevent you from safely undertaking a high intensity interval training program, start working out hard in short bursts. Always remember to warm up first for 5-10 minutes with low level activity, and then go for it with hard/easy cycles of exercise. You can do this with walking, running, on the treadmill, on the elliptical, or even in the pool.

Things to consider if your goal is weight loss

Many people come to me with a goal of wanting to see the number on their bathroom scale decrease. I completely understand this. Scale weight is a really quick and easy way to track progress. However, I always have a conversation with new clients about how the scale doesn't tell the whole story.

Here's an example:

You could have a very salty restaurant meal tonight and see 2-5 additional pounds on your bathroom scale tomorrow. On the other hand, you could have an unfortunate bout of food borne illness for the next 24 hours and be down 2-5 pounds on your bathroom scale at the end of that 24 hours. Have you gained fat with the salty restaurant meal – or lost fat with the food borne illness? No. Your salty restaurant meal made you hold more fluid which showed up as extra pounds on the scale. The bout with food borne illness made you lose fluid which dropped your scale weight.

Neither of these episodes changed the amount of fat on your body – but the scale moved in each case. Fluid changes show up on your bathroom scale but those fluid changes aren't necessarily a great indication of what's going on with the fat to muscle ratio in your body.

How do we track fat loss, then?

The best way is to have your body fat percentage measured right as you begin your journey of improving your health and fitness and monitor it at intervals thereafter. The body fat scales or hand held devices you can buy at your local store or online technically do measure your fat mass – but they're very unreliable and I don't recommend them.

If you belong to a health club where a qualified coach can measure your body fat with a skinfold caliper, this is a decent way to go to get a quick, easy measurement that is pretty accurate. If you live near a college campus that has an exercise physiology lab, they may be able to perform a hydrostatic measurement or "underwater weighing" test on you that is quite accurate. This isn't a viable or convenient option for most of us, though.

For the individual looking to lose weight, I suggest you not only track your scale weight, but that you also measure your chest, waist and hips with a flexible measuring tape. Although circumference measurements don't give you a measurement of your body fat, these measurements are one more piece of the fitness puzzle that can indicate whether or not you're making positive changes in your body.

Muscle is a dense, compact tissue that doesn't take up as much room as fat. Some people may put on a significant amount of muscle when they start exercising and they'll get frustrated if they're only looking at scale weight. They'll wonder why they aren't losing weight. Well...the bathroom scale may not be changing, but their circumference measurements likely are.

I saw this recently with a 46-year old female client who was quite frustrated that she hadn't lost as much weight as she wanted by a certain time period (she had actually lost 12 pounds in about 9 1/2 weeks of working with me—which is terrific!). We measured her body fat and did circumference measurements. The results showed that she had lost nearly 3% body fat and over 8 inches in just 5 measurements—4 inches in her waist alone. She was disappointed that she hadn't lost more scale weight. Gah! I explained to her that the strength training and interval cardio program I created and the nutrition coaching I did was geared toward muscle preservation and fat loss – and that's exactly what we accomplished.

Sometimes it's really, really hard to get over that dang scale weight. Please keep this in mind as you step into or continue your fitness journey. We folks over 40 need to maintain our muscle. Starving yourself and over-exercising will jeopardize your muscle mass and the scale will not tell you you're burning up your muscle. Scale weight alone may indicate "success" – when in reality you're losing muscle. I'm not telling you that you must throw your scale away. I'm simply suggesting that if weight loss is your goal, consider fat loss the priority and monitor a couple other fitness parameters as you measure your progress.

Setting up measurable goals

In this chapter, I've talked about the important of training for your goal. Before we close out this chapter, I think it's important that we talk about setting up goals the right way.

I'm guessing you've heard of the acronym S.M.A.R.T. with regard to goal setting. Just in case you haven't, here is what the acronym stands for:

Specific
Measurable
Attainable
Realistic
Time sensitive

Let's look at each parameter:

Specific: A goal of "I want to get healthier" (I hear that a lot, by the way) is a wonderful goal, but it's not specific. Now, saying "I want to decrease my fasting blood sugar to under "##." That is specific. Saying you want to lose "X" number of pounds is also specific.

Get specific! Give me something you, your fitness coach or your personal physician can measure.

Measurable: I can't measure "I want to eat healthier." It's a great goal, but not measurable. Tell me how eating better will look for you. Perhaps it's "I will eat a minimum of 'X' vegetable servings a day most days of the week." or "I will drink ½ my weight in ounces of water every day."

Attainable and Realistic: These two parameters can be hard for some people to figure out. If you're trying to get 6-pack abs and you never had them in your teens—it might be attainable, but it's probably not realistic for you. If you have access to an experienced fitness coach, ask him/her if your specific and measurable goals are attainable in the timeframe you've outlined.

Time Sensitive: All goals should have a date by which you will accomplish them. I usually set goals with my clients for 8-12 weeks out. If some of their goals will take longer (for instance, a large amount of scale weight loss), we reverse engineer the big goal into smaller segments that are attainable in 8-12 weeks. Once we get to the 8 to 12-week mark, we re-measure and set new goals.

One thing I notice on client goal sheets is that many of the goals they list in their first rendition of their goal sheet are what I call "process goals" instead of the outcome they want. For instance, a client may write, "I will walk three times a week and eat healthier." That's all fine and good, but that's not an outcome, that's the process by which you'll get to your specific and measurable goal.

Outcome is what you want (smaller waistline, lower blood sugar, lower body fat, increased strength).

The process is what you'll do to get it (eat less sugar, exercise 5 times a week, strength training 3 times a week, etc.).

Your Action Plan

I've given you a goal sheet in Appendix A that I use with my clients.

Use it to write out your specific and measurable goals. You'll notice that in the first line of the form, I'm asking for your outcome goals. The second line is where you'll list your process for achieving your goals.

Once completed, tear out your goal sheet and place it where you can see it.

Want additional accountability? Share your goals
(and goal dates) with a friend.

3

Rule #3: Mind Your Muscle

I truly believe that if there is such a thing as The Fountain of Youth, it can be found through strength training. In the previous chapter, I suggested that you train for the goal. You're an individual with a mind of your own, and your very own personal fitness goals. But, if you are over 40, I strongly suggest you consider adding strength training to your exercise program. I'd love for increased muscle mass to become one of your goals. It's one of my goals for you.

In the introduction, I mentioned that the concept of muscle mass decreasing with age may be more a factor of disuse than chronological age. Therefore, I just had to have one of my rules be about maintaining muscle mass. I absolutely believe that maintaining your strength will decrease your risk for falls as you age, keep you feeling younger and help you lead a more independent life as you hit your 8th and 9th decades. But it starts now. If you wait until you're frail, it's hard to catch up.

Why strength training after 40 is a MUST

Strength training maintains your muscle mass

Maintaining your muscle keeps your metabolism humming along so that you don't suffer that dreaded "metabolism slow down" as much. I'll go out on a limb and say that a great many of the over-40 crowd who don't strength train will add fat to their frame every year. Even people who look visibly slim may carry too much fat and not enough muscle on their frame if they don't strength train (in my industry, we call this "skinny fat").

A study by Harvard School of Public Health showed that healthy men who worked out with weights for just 20 minutes daily experienced less of an increase in age-related belly fat compared with men who spent the same amount of time doing aerobic activities alone. The test subjects who did both strength training and aerobic activity had the best outcomes.

So, you see, strength training isn't just about getting bigger biceps – it's about controlling overall fat gain as we age. Yes, toned arms look great, but a lean belly looks good, too. A lean belly may also help you avoid heart disease.

A well-designed strength training program keeps you functional and improves your posture

What I mean by the term functional is that you're able to bend, stretch and move your body with ease. When you're functionally strong and fit, you're able to get up off the floor, move a piece of furniture, lift your grandkids or walk up steep stairs at an arena or stadium. The more easily you can perform basic functions with your body weight, the more agile and functional (and independent) you'll be as you age.

With all my clients over 40, I use exercises that have them squat, lunge and rotate—sometimes while holding something that they have to pull or push against—so that they not only work on their strength, but also their agility, mobility and balance.

For a number of years, I've offered a specialized program twice a week just for women over 40, and I repeatedly tell that group that if they want to instantly look younger—change their posture. The same thing goes for men, too, but for some reason, I mention the posture concept to my female clients more. It really makes you look older and more haggard when your shoulders are sagging forward and your upper back is rounded. I think most of us can improve our posture simply by being aware of it (Chest open! Head up!).

I include postural exercises in my programming for every single client regardless of age (the millennials need help with their "text neck"). Better posture for those of us north of 40 means we'll move better, we won't tire as easily, we'll have healthier shoulders and, of course, we'll look better.

Strength training helps keep your bones strong

Strength training has been shown in numerous studies to slow down bone loss and to build bone in some populations. We used to think only "impact" exercises like running helped maintain or increase bone mass, but numerous studies have shown that a well-designed strength training program helps maintain bone just as well as higher impact activities. When we strength train, our muscles pull on our bones. This has been shown to be enough of a stimulus to create growth in the bone.

Strong bones are less likely to break. Strong bones age better. I believe that strength training is the antidote to painful knees, sore low backs and even sleep troubles in some people. Strength training at any age can enhance your health and well-being, but after 40 or 50 it can change your life.

Strength training keeps your metabolism humming

That decrease in metabolism we want to blame solely on our age is, in part, due to a decrease in muscle mass associated with a sedentary lifestyle. If you want to keep your metabolism humming along and improve your physique along the way, a well-designed strength training program is your ticket to a higher metabolic rate. The more muscle you have, the more calories you burn all day long.

Basic Strength Training Guidelines

Perform your strength training program 2-3 times per week

Most research indicates that strength training 3 times a week may be the ideal set up, but there is some recent research on people over 50 that has shown a 2 time a week program netted very similar results as a 3 time a week program. If you're new to strength training, start with just twice a week with at least one day in between strength training days.

Strength training doesn't have to be a time sink. A well-designed strength training program for general fitness (i.e., you're not trying to be a body builder or figure competitor) can be accomplished in 25-30 minutes per session.

Pick exercises that use large muscle groups and multiple muscles/joints

For example, I'd rather see you do a squat than a leg extension exercise on a machine. The squat uses more muscle than a leg extension exercise, it requires using your core muscles, it's functional (it mimics every day movement), and it will help you with your balance. It does require skill and good form, though, so find a qualified coach to help you learn to do non-machine exercises safely and effectively.

Stay standing

When possible, perform the majority of your exercises standing up. This will help you engage more core muscles and work on your balance as well. It's okay to start a strength training program using the seated machines at your health club. Those machines can be a decent entry into strength training. However, work toward doing some of your exercises with dumbbells and cable-based equipment that allows you to stand while strength training. You'll reap greater benefits from those exercises.

Be consistent

Consistency with strength training is crucial. You have to keep doing it to maintain results. Figure out a training schedule that works for you and stick to it. Treat your strength workout like the very important appointment that it is.

That old saying "Use It or Lose It" really is true with regard to muscle. You will have less muscle mass on you in the years to come if you don't do something to maintain it now. Lack of muscle can lead to poor balance and an increased risk of falls. In fact, lack of muscle is the leading cause of dependence in the elderly. Muscle loss is preventable. Please consider adding "increased muscle mass" to your goal sheet.

If you need a little kick start to begin a strength training program and want to learn how to decrease your workout time, I created two sample workouts for you and you'll find them in Appendix B. A word of caution: These sample workouts may or may not be suitable for you based on your current abilities and joint health at this particular time. However, I encourage you to look over the workouts even if you can't perform them right now. I would love for you to see what a well-rounded workout looks like. Most of the exercises are multi-joint exercises that use a lot of muscle. You'll push, you'll pull, and you'll use the front and back of your thighs and your rear end muscles in both sample workouts. You'll also use your core muscles. The sample workouts will take less than 45 minutes to complete (even including warm up time).

Your Action Plan:

Start a strength training program ASAP!

Check out Appendix B for my sample full-body workouts. If you don't know what the exercises are, type the exercise name into a search engine. You're likely to find an example online somewhere of every exercise I list.

Find a qualified coach if you're not sure how to start and progress your exercises safely.

Check your local recreation center for specialty classes or workshops for residents over 40.

If you live in or near San Jose, I'd love for you to reach out to me.

☐

4

Rule #4: Recovery Matters

Recovery is all about giving your muscles (and your entire body, for that matter) time to rest. If you're currently engaged in physical exercise on a regular basis, your body needs recovery time and recovery activity. Not only is it more important for an older exerciser to have recovery days, but some of us may need a longer recovery between challenging workouts. We don't bounce back as fast.

I'm an advocate of challenging workouts, but not challenging, exhausting workouts every single day. The day after a tough strength workout is actually when our muscles grow, so it's been common practice for fitness professionals to recommend an "every other day" schedule for their clients who are strength training so that there is adequate time between strength training sessions for muscle recovery and regeneration. For some of my clients, I'll even recommend two days between strength training sessions for better recovery.

So far, I've only mentioned strength training and the need for recovery. Should you have recovery days between running workouts, Pilates workouts, or Zumba? In general, I tell my clients that if an exercise session brings your muscles to a very high level of fatigue, I'd take the next day to rest from that activity. Recovery doesn't have to mean sitting on the couch, though. Recovery could mean a walk or a slow gentle swim after a hard run the day before. It could mean some gentle yoga a day after a long match of singles tennis.

How much recovery do we need?

This is somewhat of an individual question. If you'd like to see how different exercise combinations (number of days of harder exercise vs. easier exercise days and number of rest days) affect you, keep an exercise journal to monitor joint pain, fatigue, energy levels, etc. Over time, you'll find the best mix of rest days and exercise days. You'll also see how your body adapts to various types of exercise formats (high impact vs. low impact, high intensity vs. low intensity).

I suggest you look for balance in your overall fitness program. You may have some hard days of strength training, circuit training or long duration cardiovascular exercise. The following day, you simply dial back to something lower level and lower impact. Vary your routine. Vary the way your body moves, and always make sure you have time to rest and recover.

Suggested recovery methods

Yoga
Some forms of yoga can be intense (hot yoga, for instance). Find a format that relaxes you, stretches you and calms your mind. You can take a class locally or purchase a video to practice yoga at home. Start with a beginner video if you're new to yoga.

Walking

I especially like to see my clients get outside and into nature for walks. Walking in the hills, listening to the sounds of nature and seeing the views of the valley below is a great way to get some relaxing exercise in. What's more, you get some fresh air and a little Vitamin D when you walk outdoors.

Breathing Exercises

Just 10-15 minutes of stretching, deep breathing and mindfulness meditation can do wonders for rejuvenating your body and mind. You can find several apps for your phone that will help guide you in a 5 to 15-minute breathing and relaxation session.

Foam rolling

Foam rolling is an excellent way to help repair and relax your muscles. Foam rolling massages your muscles, brings blood flow to your muscles and helps break up scar tissue. You can purchase a foam roller online or at a local sporting goods store.

You can find links to a few foam rolling videos I've done in the References section at the end of this book.

Important factors concerning recovery

Sleep

Bottom line: Sleep heals. Sleep helps balance your hormones and allows your body to repair itself after an intense workout. Now, I'm not telling you to take a nap after your workout, but I am telling you that sleeping well overnight is important in the muscle recovery process.

It's probably a good idea at this juncture since we're talking about sleep to also mention that sleep is hugely important if weight loss is a goal of yours. When you don't sleep enough or you don't sleep well, your hormones can wreak havoc on your eating behavior and feelings of well-being the next day.

Two hormones that are key in this process are ghrelin and leptin. Ghrelin is the "go" hormone that tells you when to eat. When you are sleep-deprived, your body excretes more ghrelin. Leptin is the hormone that tells you to stop eating. When you are sleep deprived, researchers have found that there seems to be a problem with leptin in our system. We either have less circulating leptin when we're sleep deprived or we are more resistant to it (researchers aren't sure yet).

To make the hormone story even worse—the more sleep-deprived you are, the more your adrenal glands excrete excess cortisol. A little cortisol in your system is good, but excess cortisol from lack of sleep stokes your appetite. Research has shown that when people are sleep deprived, they reach for more processed carbohydrates (probably as an unconscious attempt to "medicate").

When you're tired, you're more likely to make food choices based on whatever is easiest and will make you feel better in that moment.

So, you see, adequate sleep is important for muscle recovery, weight management and just to feel decent during the day. When you feel lousy due to poor sleep, everything is out of whack—your eating, your exercise and your feeling of well-being. Not a good situation.

If getting good, quality sleep is a problem for you, here are some tips to help you improve your sleep:

1) Support your body's natural rhythms

-Be careful of napping too long
-Avoid sleeping in too long on weekends
-Attempt to get to bed at the same time each night

2) Control your exposure to light

-Expose yourself to natural light as soon as you can in the morning

-If you work indoors, try to work near natural light and get outdoors a few times a day

-Avoid electronic devices right before bed

-When it is time to sleep, make sure your room is dark (watch out for LED clocks)

3) Get regular exercise

-You knew I was going to say this, right?

-The more vigorous the exercise, the more sleep promoting it is

-Exercise too close to bedtime can interfere with some people's sleep, so be aware of how evening exercise affects your sleep quality

4) Be mindful of what you eat and drink

-Be careful about afternoon caffeine

-Avoid big meals late at night

-Figure out if evening alcohol disrupts your sleep in the middle of the night – it does for a lot of people

-Avoid too many liquids in the hour before you go to bed

5) Improve your sleep environment

-Optimal room temperature is 63-67 degrees
-Dim the lights in the 30 minutes leading up to bed
-Keep noise down
-Experiment with pillows, mattress toppers, etc. to
find the best bed/pillow combination

6) Wind down/clear your head

-Create bed-time ritual (yoga, stretching,
meditation, reading, aromatherapy)
-In order to clear your head of "things," write down
a to-do list for tomorrow and then let all the head
chatter go

Hydration

Most of us don't drink enough water. Water is not
only extremely important in the muscle recovery
process, but also to help you feel good and perform
well during your day.

I went to a lecture many years ago where the
Registered Dietician who was speaking (a woman to
whom I still refer my clients to this day) told the

audience that a very large percentage of people who came to her complained of fatigue and mild headaches. She said, "This isn't a nutrition problem, folks. This is quite likely a hydration problem in a great number of these people."

Well, geez. There's a simple fix for this. Drink more water daily.

The best advice I can give you here is to start your day with a glass of water. Yep, even before your cup of coffee. To be better hydrated daily, start tomorrow off by drinking a glass of water as soon as you awaken.

Since we were kids, most of us have heard the suggestion to "drink 8 glasses of water a day." I suppose that's an adequate suggestion, but wouldn't people of different sizes need different amounts of water each day? For instance, a man who is 6'4" and 220 pounds likely needs more fluids than a woman who is 4' 11" and 100 pounds.

I tell my clients that a good rule of thumb is to drink ½ your weight in ounces. So, if you weigh 150 pounds, your goal would be to drink 75 ounces of water a day. One way to tell if you're getting enough water is to check the color of your urine. If you are well hydrated, your urine should be very pale yellow (assuming you aren't taking any medications that change the color of your urine). If it's not, you might need to drink more water.

I often hear from clients that they get bored with "just drinking water." I get it. It's not that exciting. But you still need to do it. Try to liven things up a bit by squeezing some lemon or lime in your water on occasion, or having some carbonated water every now and then.

If you can't remember to drink water, there's an app for that. You'll find several apps to choose from at the app store on your smartphone.

No excuses. Get in the habit of drinking more water if you don't currently drink enough. I promise you, you'll feel better and you'll be helping your body recover from exercise more efficiently. Cool bonus side-effect of drinking more water: You might even lose a little weight.

Sometimes when you're feeling the urge to put food in your mouth, your body is really telling you it needs some fluid. So, the next time you feel like eating, but your stomach isn't growling, drink some water instead. Your pants may fit a little better in a few weeks just by this little habit change.

Stress Management

We all have stressful moments, days or events in our lives. It's part of being human. However, chronic stress is not okay. Chronic stress is not healthy. Chronic stress can accelerate certain disease processes, suppress the immune system, and it makes full recovery from hard exercise very difficult.

When we're in a state of chronic stress, our body just can't fully recover. If your body can't fully recover, you aren't able to heal your muscles. What's more, if you're chronically stressed, you're probably not eating or sleeping well. If you're chronically stressed, your blood sugar and/or blood pressure could be elevated which puts your overall health at risk.

Remember, when we're over 40, we don't bounce back as well. Managing stress and staying well takes daily, consistent effort.

Just like poor sleep quality, high levels of stress can create health problems; weight loss resistance being one of them. If you are stressed, seek out ways to learn to manage it. Sometimes we can't totally remove sources of stress in our life (they could be people we love!), but we certainly can find ways to manage stressful situations and find new ways to react to them.

Many people find Yoga, T'ai Chi or meditation helpful for managing stress. Others find that keeping a gratitude journal helps with stress levels. Try some different stress management techniques and see what works for you.

As you learn to manage stress, your cortisol levels will come down. Lower levels of cortisol could mean better sleep, less inflammation and better blood sugar or blood pressure readings. All these things will create an environment that supports recovery from exercise.

Your Action Plan

If you are currently physically active, assess your average weekly routine. Does it include adequate recovery? If not, develop a plan of action to include recovery days and/or recovery activities into your schedule moving forward.

Check your current sleep/wake patterns over the next week. How many hours are you averaging a night? If it's less than 7, devise a plan to begin to increase sleep time in small increments over the next few weeks. This might mean changing your evening routines a bit. I know change is hard, but please don't skip this step. If you're getting less than 7 hours nightly or you're waking up a lot during the night and not falling back to sleep—this can lead to health problems. Make quality sleep a top priority.

Calculate your average water intake over the next few days. Are you getting about half your weight in ounces every day? If not, make an effort to change this.

If chronic stress is getting the best of you, make a pact with yourself to put stress management at the top of your list. Chronic stress affects many systems in your body. It can age you and make you sick. Get an action plan together to bring your stress levels down. Look for a mindfulness meditation class (and, yes, there is an app for mindfulness, too). Sign up for a yoga class. Talk things out with a counselor.

5

Rule #5: Be Flexible

Now that you've hit or passed the 40-year mark, I'd like you to think of flexibility in a couple of ways.

The first form of flexibility relates to your body and how it moves. Maintaining flexibility and mobility in your joints and muscles as you age is extremely important. Ideally, some form of flexibility/mobility work needs to be part of your exercise routine.

The second form of flexibility relates to your mind and how you approach aging and the changes your body goes through. I encourage you to be flexible and supple in your approach to aging. Have a flexible mindset, if you will.

Let's take a deeper look at both of these concepts:

Maintain a flexible physique

I encourage you to make sure to include movement or exercise in your daily routine that keeps your muscles and joints limber. Flexibility is high on the list of attributes that will keep you agile and pain free as you age. If you allow your body to get stiff and immobile, it will eventually make movement painful. With lack of movement, well...we've already established that this can lead you down a slippery slope to poor health and dependence on others. I don't want that to happen to you.

Do you feel as limber as you did when you were 25? Before we decide that "we're old, and that's just the way it goes," let's re-visit that question I brought up in the introduction about whether these changes are due to aging or due to lack of use.

My personal experience is that most sedentary folks over 40 will tell me they feel stiff and slow. In contrast, the active exercisers I know, even though they may have several arthritic joints, move better, feel better and report less pain.

Why is this?

I believe it's because the active adults have better joint mobility, better muscular flexibility and stronger muscles than their sedentary counterparts. They're just keeping their parts well-oiled.

Now, many folks over 40 will attribute stiff, sore joints to arthritis. Yes, arthritis happens, and it might be happening in you. I've got several joints that are arthritic myself. Feeling stiff isn't just about arthritis, though. It's about tight muscles, inflexible tendons and dried out joints.

We can't get rid of arthritis once we have it (the structure of your joint has changed), but we can do something about tight muscles, inflexible tendons and less lubricated joints – we can maintain our flexibility.

Current research on arthritis supports the notion that exercising for strength and flexibility helps manage arthritis pain. We know that regular exercise improves strength and that specifically working your joints through ranges of motion that stretch them improves your mobility. What's more, some studies find that exercise decreases the pain of arthritis better than medication (and exercise doesn't hurt your liver like some medications can!).

The added benefit of exercise is that while it's making you stronger and more flexible, it improves your joint range of motion, your balance, and a whole lot of other things drugs can't do for you. Arthritis is a physical change at the joint that can't be reversed— but we can work toward decreasing the pain, inflammation and stiffness associated with it.

So, what should we do to feel more flexible and maintain our joint range of motion? Next to strength training, one of the best ways to decrease your feeling of muscular stiffness or to decrease the pain of arthritis is to stretch. If there's one area of overall fitness that I've come to respect a lot more as I've gotten older, it's stretching and using my foam roller to roll out muscle tension. Older muscles just need a little more care and feeding in order to perform well and recover well.

For best results, I have my clients work on flexibility at the end of their workout. Their muscles are warm, their tendons and joints are more lubricated and therefore their bodies are more receptive to the stretches I put them through.   Stretching is also a wonderful way to close out a great exercise session.

What's the best way to stretch?

Although I'm a proponent of stretching after an exercise session for the reasons I just mentioned, I'm also a proponent of having you plan your flexibility exercises when you're most likely to do them consistently. Stretching can be a great way to start your day. I have a few clients who report that they love to do some gentle stretches (knee to chest, for instance) when they're still in bed in the morning.

Jan B., one of my dear clients for over 14 years told me that her back felt so much better the whole day if she did a few "knees to chest" and "knees to each side" while she lay in bed in the morning. It was a great way for her to warm up her back muscles and stretch her hip muscles before her feet hit the floor each morning. One of the key reasons this benefitted Jan was because she did this consistently. Every. Single. Day. If she did by chance miss a day, she didn't feel as limber.

I like to have my clients over the age of 40 pay special attention to their lower body (hips, legs and ankles), spine and shoulders when they're stretching. I do an assessment with each client when I first start working with them so that I can make sure to address any specific muscular tightness or joint mobility issues they may have. I then program some "fixes" into their exercise program to help get them more flexible or mobile exactly where they need it.

To get you started on a general flexibility/mobility program you can do anywhere (no gym required), I made some short videos to teach you some gentle stretching and mobility exercises. You can find the links to the videos in the References section at the end of this book.

Making an effort to maintain or improve our flexibility doesn't have to take hours a day. Minutes a day will suffice. I'm all for time-efficiency, so I usually sneak mobility and flexibility work right into my client's program. This way, each time they come to see me, I'm able to help them get a little bit more limber. You can do the same thing with your personal strength or cardio workouts. Stretch between strength sets. Do some stretches after a run on the treadmill or after a hike in the hills. That old adage of "Use It Or Lose It" really rings true when it comes to our flexibility.

My wish for you is to move your body a little bit every day. The days you don't do a dedicated strength or cardio workout are ideal days to work on flexibility. I suggest that all my clients stretch and do foam rolling on their rest days. It's a great gift to your hardworking muscles.

I think we can agree our muscles and joints are not the same as they were in when we were in our 20's, but with a small amount of consistent, daily effort, you can keep your body limber and flexible for many years to come.

Not only will you move better with some daily attention to flexibility, I believe you're going to feel better as well.

Maintain a flexible mindset

Our bodies really do change in our 4th and 5th decades and beyond. What worked for us when we were 30 might not be the best approach to staying fit and healthy in our 40's. I want to encourage you to be okay with change. Please understand, I am not asking you to settle and do less because you're getting "old." I'm asking you to be open to listening to your body and being willing to do things differently if it yields a better result.

Here's an example:

My client, Patrick (not his real name), is a 58-year old software engineer who is a very accomplished cyclist. He's been cycling for many years and it brings him a great deal of enjoyment to get out and ride. Not to mention it keeps him in great shape. He began to have more knee pain and began to wonder if his cycling days were over. We started including additional hip strengthening exercises and more thigh stretches and foam rolling into his routine, but he also manipulated how he planned his rides. He found that if he started a ride and quickly went uphill, his knee hurt more. If he had a longer time on flat ground before going uphill – he had less knee pain. I believe his body simply needed a longer warm up before his knee could successfully handle the uphill push without pain. He didn't need to quit cycling or even cycle less. Patrick simply needed a longer warm up. He figured out what his body needed, made some adjustments to his cycling routine and continued on his health and fitness journey. Rather than decide he couldn't do something, he figured out what he could do. Problem solved.

There will be times when you find you can't do something the way that you used to and it and it will be really frustrating. This is totally normal. Rather than give up—take a flexible approach and figure out what you *can* do like Patrick did.

Your Action Plan

Commit to adding some sort of flexibility training into your routine. This can be as simple as a 5-minute stretch most days of the week, or a yoga class added into your week somewhere.

Be aware of your self-talk or your biases around aging. We all make "I'm getting old jokes" once in a while and laugh at ourselves. That's normal. But— don't let an inflexible mindset keep you from trying to improve. It doesn't matter what your age or fitness level is at this moment while you read this. You can improve and get better. Be mindful of your concepts on aging and your own personal abilities. Avoid settling for less than you can achieve. You are different than the generations that came before you.

6

Rule #6: You Can't Out Train a Poor Diet

Many people come to me thinking that if they just hire a fitness coach and exercise 2-3 times a week then everything will fall into place. They believe exercise alone will get them to their fitness goals. Don't shoot the messenger, but that's not how it works.

If fat loss is your goal, we simply have to talk about what you're eating. What you eat will absolutely, positively shape (quite literally) what you look like. In fact, even if getting stronger or faster is your goal and you aren't trying to decrease body fat, we should still be talking about food. Your nutrition not only affects your waistline, but it also affects your physical performance. Good nutrition, or lack thereof, will also affect your overall well-being and risk for certain diseases.

So, yes, my friend, we have to talk about nutrition if I'm going to help you live your fittest life ever.

You see, if I can help you navigate the non-workout hours of your week (e.g., eat well, sleep well, manage stress well), I'm going to help you create a healthier, leaner more productive body. I like to call this "coaching you through the other 165+ hours" of your week. How you manage your life in those non-workout hours of the week will have a profound effect on your overall health and well-being as you move past the age of 40.

I suspect for you, as it is for most of my clients, the "other 165 hours" in your week will center around what's in your kitchen (and to some extent what's at your workplace) and social events. This reminds me of a popular meme that circulates on the internet now and again that says something like "flat abs are made in the kitchen." I'd add that decreasing your risk for disease and, in some cases, even less pain from arthritis begins in the kitchen.

Food can kill you or food can heal you.

So, what diet should a person over 40 follow?

If you learn anything from me by reading this book, please learn this:

Don't ever start another "diet" again!

Allow me to offer you my definition of "diet" so that we're on the same page here.

I define a "diet" as a restrictive eating regimen that you undertake in order to lose weight quickly. It often severely restricts calories or eliminates complete food groups or food types. A "diet" is something that you would find very hard to stay with for the long term due to the restrictive nature of it. A "diet" is temporary.

If you're over 40, you've been around long enough to experience tons of different diets.

- The cabbage soup diet
- The cookie diet
- The liquid diet
- The Zone Diet
- Atkins Diet
- The South Beach Diet
- The Blood Type Diet

Phew. That's just off the top of my head. I'm sure there are more that you've tried or heard of. It can be really, really confusing to make sense of all the nutrition information out there.

Some of the diets I listed actually do a good job of moving you toward eating more "real" foods and fewer non-nutritious, highly processed foods. That's a good thing.

Here's the problem with diets, though.

You eventually go off of them.

This chapter is all about getting away from the diet mindset and taking a different approach to learning how to eat for better health and a smaller waistline. We'll start by going over some basic guidelines for eating healthfully and then I'll help you with a plan to begin implementing the guidelines. Information is great, but unless you take action on the information, it does you no good. So, I'll be giving you some step-by-step ideas on how to implement what you learn here.

One of the themes that I remind my clients of often is the "80/20 rule." I let them know that I don't expect rigid perfection with regard to nutrition. I am by no means perfect in my nutrition. I don't expect my clients or you to be either. What I expect is that you put effort into eating better over time, most of the time. If you can eat really well 80 percent of the time, the other 20 percent doesn't matter. This is what I'd like you to keep in mind as you read through the rest of the chapter. The idea of "80/20" should help you not feel deprived or label certain foods or food behaviors as bad. We can consider some foods/food behaviors as "once in a while" things.

What often happens when you try a new diet or you pledge to "start eating healthy on Monday," is that your current lifestyle doesn't support the changes that the diet you've chosen requires. You may have too many triggers at work, at home, or in your social life that make that diet hard to maintain. Therefore, over time, the diet goes away because it's tiring and/or stressful to maintain.

So, if I'm asking you to never, ever diet again...what the heck do I want you to do?

I want you to consider moving toward healthier eating over time. No quick fixes. No massive restrictions.

In a nutshell, here's what I'd suggest you do to begin eating healthier (we'll get into more details later):

- Eat real, whole, minimally processed foods most of the time

- Minimize how much food you eat that is made with refined wheat flour

- Increase the amount of fresh vegetables you eat daily

- Increase the amount of water you drink daily

- Add some healthy fats to your daily eating plan

- Decrease the amount of added sugar you eat

Now, if those bullet points up there are a far cry from where you are now, by all means, don't try to do all of those things up there tomorrow. Pick one of those bullet points and work on it for a few weeks until it becomes a habit. Then pick another change from the list above to work on.

By eating mostly whole, unprocessed food, you'll fill up on high fiber, highly nutritious, highly satiating food. Eating high quality food is important for good health and energy levels, muscle building and brain function. Another bonus of eating real, whole food:

The more real food you eat, the less junk you tend to eat over time.

You won't find an actual meal plan in this book because I believe that everyone's body/body chemistry is slightly different. What works to make one person feel great and function at their best may be different for someone else. Some people may do better on an eating plan that's a little higher in protein and fat and a little lower in carbohydrates. Another person might feel better and perform better with slightly higher carbohydrates and not as much fat and protein. My goal with this chapter is to give you some basics on what to do nutritionally to eat a sustainable healthy diet that will help fuel you for activity/exercise, decrease your risk for disease and help you lose excess weight if you need to.

I tell all my clients that I do not expect perfection from them with their nutrition. I simply expect progress.

By focusing on the quality and quantity of the food you eat and tuning in to how certain foods make you feel, you'll begin to see patterns and potentially discover certain foods just don't agree with you.

So what should you do?

Let's start by going into a little more depth on the 6 principles I listed earlier.

Eat real, whole, minimally processed foods most of the time

The closer your food is how it was naturally grown, the better. Now, of course, we all know there is no such thing as a "meat tree" and I am not asking you to eat like a caveman. I think we can all agree that if we eat animal protein that we didn't hunt and kill ourselves, it has been rendered and packaged for us. Some processing has been involved. Same thing for dairy. What I'm suggesting here is to eat foods that are as close to their original form as possible. Avoid Frankenfoods that have no resemblance to the whole food item from which they were made (think: Cheetos or Doritos).

Examples of whole, minimally processed foods:

Fresh beef, chicken, turkey, fish and shellfish
Fresh fruits and vegetables
Eggs
Beans, lentils, peas
Raw nuts
Natural nut butters (no sugar added)
Whole grains: Bulgar, barley, farro, oats, brown
rice, quinoa (technically a seed)
**Plain Greek yogurt
Grass fed butter

**Yes, it's processed to some degree but healthy for
you if there's no added sugar in it.

Aside from providing you with vitamins and
minerals, another reason a diet high in whole,
minimally processed foods is so important is that
these foods fill you up. These types of foods are not
only high in nutrition, they're often high in fiber.
Fiber helps keep you feeling full. Foods high in
healthy fats (olives, avocados, and nuts) help you feel
full as well.

When you are satiated and your blood sugar is
steady, you feel great and will be less likely to binge

on junk food. A well-nourished body just doesn't crave the junk as much.

Minimize how much food you eat that is made with refined wheat flour

What I'm referring to here are things like breads, cookies, crackers, cakes, pastries traditional pasta and muffins. Please know I am not asking you never to eat a piece of bread or a cookie again. What I do want you to know is that many people make this "food group" the majority of their diet. That's what I want you to avoid. A diet high in refined, processed grains is likely putting many people at risk for disease (obesity, high blood sugar, and heart disease to name a few). I don't want that to be you. I'd like you to take note of how much food you eat on a daily basis that is made from refined, bleached wheat flour. Probably more than you think.

Let's take a closer look at a refined grain product versus a whole food product. I'm sure you can appreciate the difference between eating a cup of fresh strawberries versus eating a strawberry Pop-Tart. It doesn't take a genius to know one is a little closer to nature than the other. The Pop-Tart has been processed and combined with other foods (and non-foods). The nutrition that was available to you in the fresh strawberries is gone. I'm not actually sure if there even is any real strawberry in a strawberry Pop Tart. The pastry has artificial flavors, colors, and added sugar. There is no nutrition for you in this food item whatsoever. Now, some of my clients who like to be a little sarcastic would say, "Awwww, but Coach Becky, the strawberry Pop-Tart tastes soooooo much better!" I hear that a lot about a processed food tasting better than a whole, unprocessed food. The sad thing is, our taste buds have gotten accustomed to fake foods.

Here's where eating a lot of processed, highly refined carbohydrates can get problematic: They're messing with your hormones. Take the example of that Pop-Tart. It's made with lots of sugar and chemicals, plus refined white flour. Because this little food item is highly refined and processed, it's sort of been pre-digested for you. When you eat it, it's broken down and digested very quickly which raises your blood sugar very quickly. When your blood sugar spikes, your brain tells your pancreas to excrete a lot of insulin because it's not good to have a high level of sugar in your blood. Your pancreas does its job and the insulin shuttles sugar out of your bloodstream and into your muscles for storage. But because the spike of sugar in your blood was fast, the shot of insulin was large and your blood sugar will now come down quickly which can lead to low blood sugar symptoms: crankiness, hunger and sometimes jitters and irritability. Guess what you reach for when this happens? Yep, you guessed it. That other Pop-Tart in the dang package. Processed foods that are digested quickly and high in refined grains really mess with your appetite, your energy level, your mood and your waistline.

Had you chosen the fresh strawberries, you would have had a high fiber, high nutrition snack with a very different blood sugar response. Foods with naturally occurring sugar and fiber (think fruits and veggies) are digested more slowly than highly refined, non-fibrous foods that have a lot of added sugar in them. The slower the digestion, the slower the rise in blood sugar, the lower the insulin level. Research tells us that chronically high circulating insulin levels in your blood can lead to serious health problems.

Bottom line: Highly refined and processed fast digesting grain-based foods may make you crave more of the same. They can cause wild highs and lows with your blood sugar. Work on making them a much smaller part of your daily food choices.

Minimize how many calories you drink

This is one of the first things I work on with clients who come to me wanting to lose fat. I look at their food journals to see how many calories they're drinking. Liquid calories add up fast and they don't really register in your brain or stomach as food – but they can add inches to your waistline.

One of the worst types of liquids you can drink is a beverage with added sugar. I'm not just talking soda pop here. Commercially prepared orange juice is full of added sugar. Those tasty coffee drinks you get at your local coffee shop? Loaded with added sugar. We've already established what happens when you eat a food (or in this case, drink a liquid) that is digested quickly. It raises your blood sugar quickly. Trust me, that soda or that mocha from the coffee shop is hitting your blood stream fast. Drink high sugar liquids enough and you're going to add inches to your waistline.

The other sinister thing our sweet drinks are doing is fostering our sweet tooth. So, even the sugar free drinks are at odds with our healthy eating habits. They're feeding the need for "sweet."

What to do? Save that glass of orange juice for an occasional breakfast out, and go somewhere where they serve fresh squeezed juice (no added sugar). If you love coffee drinks, treat yourself to a mocha once or twice a month instead of once a day. If you drink drip coffee in the morning and like it sweetened, add less sweetener to your morning coffee. Over time, your taste buds will adapt and you'll prefer a coffee that's less sweet.

If you drink alcohol, I'm not going to ask you to stop altogether. I will ask you to be aware of how much you drink, though. Some people I know have really big wine glasses. Was that really one glass of wine last night—or more like 16 ounces? It adds up, my friend. If you're looking to slim down your waistline or drop a few pounds and you drink alcohol daily—start cutting back.

The best beverages for people wishing to be leaner: filtered water and brewed green tea. If water bores you, add sliced lemons or limes. Switch to carbonated water to change things up.

Increase the amount of fresh vegetables you eat

Most of us don't eat enough. Calorie for calorie, veggies are nutritional powerhouses. You get health-promoting vitamins, minerals, fiber and antioxidants from vegetables. If you can, eat them fresh and organic. Next best is frozen. Just be careful when you choose frozen veggies that you avoid products with added flavorings and sauces. Your food is getting more processed when other junk is added in.

If you can eat a large salad at lunch every day or a side salad with your evening meal, this is a good way to get some good produce into your eating plan each day. Eating veggie based snacks is another way to increase your daily veggie intake. Good ideas for veggie snacks include mini carrots or sweet red pepper strips dipped in hummus or celery with natural peanut butter (or almond or cashew butter). One of my favorite side dishes for a winter dinner is a mound of roasted veggies. I simply drizzle a little olive oil over mixed, chopped veggies on a sheet pan, season with salt, pepper and garlic powder and roast for 35-40 minutes. Roasted veggies are delicious and nutritious and they make great left overs the next day for lunch.

Here are some sneakier ways to increase your fresh veggie intake:

- Substitute "riced" cauliflower for the rice in stir fry recipes
- Substitute zucchini "noodles" for pasta in pasta dishes
- Add some left-over veggies from dinner into a morning omelet or egg scramble
- Add sautéed veggies (red pepper, kale, mushrooms) to prepared pasta sauce
- Throw some spinach or kale into a morning protein shake

It is recommended that we eat 6-9 servings of vegetables a day. I know this sounds like a lot. However, a large salad (about 2-3 cups of greens) with chopped veggies in it will provide about 3-4 servings of veggies depending on the volume of chopped veggies you add to your salad.

Increase the amount of water you drink daily

I covered this in an earlier chapter, but it bears repeating here in our nutrition section. If you're not currently drinking about ½ ounce of water for every pound of your body weight daily, begin increasing your intake. Your body will be happier with more fluids. A side benefit to increasing your water intake is that over time it could change some of your eating behaviors that cause you to gain weight.

Add some healthy fats to your daily eating plan

If you grew up in the 70's or 80's, you grew up in a time when just about all dietary fat got demonized. We were told that the fats in our food were giving us heart disease and high cholesterol. Fat was making us fat and sick, news reports told us. Food manufacturers started making fat-free versions of lots of different food items and we gobbled them up. We ate fat free cookies, fat free salad dressings, fat free yogurt, and fat free milk. But not many of us got any leaner or healthier.

Unfortunately, with many food products when you take fat out, you lose flavor. So manufacturers added back flavor with refined sugar, artificial flavors and salt. This did nothing for our health and gave us a taste for highly processed, quickly digested foods. Remember, when food is quickly digested it can lead to spikes in blood sugar. Fat and protein slow down digestion and make blood sugar rise more slowly. When you pull 100% of the fat out, the blood sugar response is different. What's more, dietary fat helps with many digestive processes, like helping us absorb nutrients. If we don't eat some dietary fat, we don't always absorb all the goodness from the fresh fruits and veggies we eat.

By asking you to be okay with adding fat to your diet, I'm not asking you to throw caution to the wind and eat gobs of butter, bacon and ribeye steaks on a daily basis. I just want to make sure you know that healthy fats in your daily diet are important and they're good for you. Toss the fat-free products. Eat healthy fat in moderation.

Here's what I suggest with respect to healthy fats in your diet:

- If you have non-fat dairy (yogurt, cheese or milk) or non-fat salad dressing at home, get rid of them and re-stock with low fat versions.

- Discard fat free peanut butter and use natural peanut butter with just salt and peanuts on the ingredient list.

- Use real (preferably grass fed) butter in moderation instead of margarine.

- For cooking, use coconut oil in moderation

- Use olive oil or walnut oil for home-made salad dressing and for roasted veggies

- Use avocados in sandwiches and salads to add healthy fat and flavor to your meal

- Enjoy raw nuts in moderation as a snack

Decrease the amount of added sugar you eat

I've listed this one last, but it is by no means the least important. In fact, next to decreasing the calories you drink, I think this is the one place many of my clients can make huge improvements in their daily eating. I'm guessing you can, too.

I think it's important to point out that I want you to be a sleuth and find out where in your normal eating plan there is added sugar. There is naturally occurring sugar in many healthy foods, and I don't want you to be worried about that.

Natural sugar is found in whole, unprocessed foods. These include fruits, vegetables, and dairy. Fructose is a natural sugar found in fruit. Lactose is a natural sugar found in animal dairy products.

Added sugar is found in processed foods and drinks. Added sugar also includes the sugar you add to foods at home (adding sugar to your coffee or your morning cereal). Added sugar provides little to no nutritional value. In processed foods, it is used for different reasons, such as:

- to keep baked goods fresh longer
- to keep jellies and jams from spoiling
- to help fermentation in breads
- to improve the flavor, color, or texture of foods and drinks

To be honest, it's likely you don't even realize how much added sugar you're eating because it's added to so many things we eat. Added sugar is in baked goods, whole wheat bread, fruit yogurt, salad dressings, barbeque sauces, fruit juices, and of course the blended coffee drinks I talked about earlier.

I really want you to get a handle on how much added sugar you're eating. Decreasing your added sugar will decrease your waistline over time and quite honestly decrease your risk for certain diseases over time. Yes, it is *that* important you do a sugar audit. If you want to feel great as you age, doing a sugar audit is a great first step in your new "I'm going to get healthier" plan.

So, first off, let's talk about how you find where hidden sugars are in the foods you eat.

You're going to need to look at the labels on the packaged food you eat. If you get a coffee drink or a muffin from a chain coffee house, look up nutrition information on the company website.

Under the ingredients list on a food label, you'll look for sugar. Oh, but you need to know that sugar in the commercial food industry goes by many names. Here are just a few other names for sugar on those labels you're going to start reading:

- agave syrup
- brown sugar
- cane juice and cane syrup
- confectioner's sugar
- corn sweetener and corn syrup
- dextrose
- fructose

- fruit juice concentrates
- glucose
- granulated white sugar
- high-fructose corn syrup
- honey
- invert sugar
- lactose
- maltose
- malt syrup
- molasses
- raw sugar
- sucrose

Yikes. I know that's a lot to remember. Do your best and start reading the labels of all the foods you eat. If "sugar" or one of the other names I've listed is one of the first three to five ingredients, you may have a high sugar item on your plate.

Keep in mind that there are naturally occurring sugars in some packaged foods that are still healthy for you. For instance, a 15 ounce can of diced tomatoes or an 8 ounce can of tomato sauce with no added sugar will show about 3 grams of sugar on the label. That's from the naturally occurring sugar in the tomatoes. If you want to find out if that can has added sugar, read the ingredient list next.

When you shop for marinara sauce, a common food that will have a significant amount of added sugar, look for a sauce with the lowest sugar count you can find. Better yet, look for one with a label that says "no sugar added." Even better, make your own sauce.

Cow's milk products (yogurt and milk) will also show a few grams of sugar on their labels. Plain yogurt will likely have about 6 or 7 grams of sugar per 8-ounce cup. That's the naturally occurring sugar (lactose) in the milk. When you see an 8-ounce cup of fruit yogurt that has 21 grams of sugar per serving, you know that roughly 14 or 15 of those grams are added sugar. Ick. Stick with plain yogurt and add fruit for sweetness.

The more you read labels and ingredient lists, the more you can begin to find the hidden sugar in your diet and begin to make changes.

Key steps to creating better eating habits

Now that we've gone over some specific areas to improve your nutrition, let's talk about how you actually make it happen.

It's one thing to know what to do.

It's another thing to actually do it.

I've seen it time and again where a new client gets really excited about working on improving their nutrition, but they fall off the wagon after a few weeks. Intuitively, they understand what to do, but they have a hard time executing consistently.

I find that failure to execute consistently usually happens due to a few common themes:

1) Changing too much too rapidly
2) Failing to plan or think ahead
3) Maintaining a non-supportive environment
4) Being unaware of food triggers

I'm guessing you may have gotten hung up with one or more of these situations as well.

I'll list below some solutions to each of these 4 habit change hold ups.

Work on ONE change at a time

As I mentioned earlier, my experience coaching hundreds of people over the years is that too much change all at once is just too stressful. It's that diet mentality where you decide that come next Monday, everything is going to change. For most of us, all that change is unsustainable. Having to think about and focus on all those different things you need to change is downright stressful and fatiguing.

Rather than change everything all at once, I coach my clients to work on one change at a time. It's not as fatiguing. Now, you're not going to lose 20 pounds in three weeks doing it this way. However, doing one change at a time, you're likely to end up with a sustainable new lifestyle habit down the road instead of one more failed diet.

I work with my clients to choose one habit change that will likely net the best outcome for the client as well as choose the habit that the client is most likely to stick with. Once we've made significant progress on making that habit part of their lifestyle, we move on to another habit to improve.

What I'd like you to do so that you don't fall into the "too much too soon" trap, is to evaluate what is one thing you can do to improve your overall nutrition starting tomorrow. Work on that and only that for the next month. That one thing will be your only focus. You don't have to be perfect at it in order to be successful, but I want you to be mindful of it every day. Focus on implementing that one habit daily.

Once it's become easier to maintain that habit and you're confident you can, challenge yourself to work on implementing another new habit.

Become a food planner

You've likely heard a quote that goes something like "Failing to plan is planning to fail." This is very true with regard to your efforts to improve your eating habits. Case in point: If you want to eat healthier, you'll need to have healthy choices in the house. That takes planning. If you come home hungry from a long day away from home and there is nothing healthy to eat for dinner, it's likely you'll make some unhealthy choices.

With a little advance planning, you can be sure to have healthy options in your home or work environment. If you can prep a few things ahead of time, it makes for quick meal preparation during the week. I often make a large, undressed salad on Sundays and use portions of it over the next few days. I'll add protein (grilled chicken strips, garbanzo beans, hard boiled eggs or left over flank steak) to a large serving of salad for lunch, or dish out a smaller serving of salad as a side with dinner. If you like to cook, plan a few weeknight dinners, shop for the ingredients on the weekend and you'll be all set to make a meal at the end of a busy work day. When I shop on the weekends, I also buy enough ingredients to make extra servings so that I can use leftovers for lunch the next day.

If you work in an office with unhealthy food options, it's important that you bring in your own healthy options. This includes snack foods as well. If you have your own healthy snacks (examples: raw nuts, plain Greek yogurt, carrots and hummus), you're less likely to dive into the donuts in the break room.

Bottom line on planning: If you want to start eating healthier, have healthier food at home and at work.

Create an environment that supports healthy eating

Your environment has a lot to do with how successful you are at any type of change. If you have chips, candies, cookies and scones in your house, it's not a supportive environment if you're trying to improve your health and eating habits. Same thing for your work environment. If you go to certain events on a regular basis (for instance, you have season tickets to a sporting event) and have a tradition of eating something unhealthy at the game, this will sabotage your efforts at being a healthier person simply due to the sheer number of times you go to your sporting event. If you attend sporting events only on occasion, enjoy your indulgence. If you're attending numerous times a season, your tradition needs to change.

Take stock of your environment and social cues. Do they support healthy eating, or cause your healthy eating efforts to go sideways? I think most of us, if we take time to observe when and where we get derailed from healthy eating, can see where our weak links are. For some of us it's work related (the candy on your co-worker's desk), for some of us it's more socially related (you spend time with people who eat and drink to excess). I'm not asking you to quit your job or stop spending time with certain friends, but I am suggesting that you'll need to take stock of what's happening in these situations and find solutions to make your environment more supportive for healthy eating.

One solution I suggest for all of my clients is to keep junk food out of the house. When it's time to enjoy an indulgence (that other 20%), go out for the indulgence instead of bringing it into your house. Make a trip out for the very best scoop of ice cream in town. Enjoy it, and then go home. A home clear of junky, processed foods is a home where someone trying to improve their eating habits has a fighting chance of doing so.

Know your food triggers

Food triggers are things (situations, emotions, events or even people) that cause you to eat unhealthy. For many people, emotional stress is a trigger to eat. For adults raising young children or grandchildren, the simple act of cleaning up their dinner plates can be a trigger to eat their left-over food. Sadness or boredom can trigger some people to eat in order to fill the void.

How do you manage these food triggers that cause you to lose control? To use a sports analogy, the best defense is a good offense. Know and understand your opponent (in this case, your food triggers). Understand how and why they come up. What makes you reach for poor food choices? Is it stress? Family situations? Boredom or sadness? Once you have an understanding of your food triggers, you have completed the first step in gaining control over them and you can begin "re-wiring" your response to situations that cause you to make poor food choices.

The power of the food journal

While we're on the subject of knowing food triggers and being mindful of our environment... Do you really know what you're eating on a daily basis?

I dare say...you may not. Research shows that our food recall isn't all that great. What's more, studies show our estimation of the portions we eat is even farther off course. I don't need to look up research to see if this is true, though. I see it in my own coaching practice all the time.

I meet with all prospective clients before bringing them into our coaching programs. I like to learn about the prospect and understand their goals and expectations to see if we're a good fit. I ask a lot of questions.

In our conversations, I often hear some variation of this story from a prospect:

"I eat a healthy diet. It's just the exercise I can't seem to get moving on."

When I hear this, I know that if we take this prospect on as a client, lots of education will be in order and I will be asking for a 5-day food journal very early in the relationship. When I get a food journal back from a client who tells me during their consultation that they eat healthy, I usually find out the client's diet isn't as healthy as they think. Sometimes it's a portion issue. The client doesn't realize how much they're really eating/drinking. Sometimes is a quality issue. The client is eating poor quality, highly processed foods that may be disrupting their blood sugar and their hormones.

I encourage you to pull out a notebook and begin to log everything you eat and drink for the next 5 days. Everything. If you're like most people, you'll find a few surprises along the way ("I ate how many Girl Scout Thin Mints over the last week?"). Earlier in this chapter, I gave you 6 guidelines on how you can improve your current diet. Compare your 5-day food journal against these 6 guidelines. Where are you doing well? Where are you way off course?

Journaling for a few days and then setting up a course of action to improve your nutrition starting with only one change that you work on consistently is my suggestion for beginning to eat healthier. This is exactly what I do with all new lifeSport Fitness personal training clients. If I help them understand basic tenants of healthy eating and then choose one thing to work on first—we end up over time with a person who has better habits and makes better choices. No crazy diets needed. They have experienced a lifestyle change. When you change your habits and your lifestyle, you can truly change the course of your life.

I hope you'll try this approach. I believe you'll find that making small, daily efforts toward getting just a little bit better beats a restrictive diet any day.

Remember...

Progress, not perfection.

Your Action Plan

Do a 5-day food journal and look for liquid calories, processed wheat flour foods, added sugar and the amount of fresh fruits and vegetables you eat.

Pick one thing (yep...just one) that you'd like to work on and improve. In some cases, this may be avoiding something (like dialing back on your soda habit) or it may be adding something (like more eating more vegetables daily). Write this one thing down on your goal sheet as one of the things you'll do to reach your goals. Work on it for one month.

When you feel yourself slipping off track on your new habit, re-visit your "Finding Your Why" worksheet and start journaling your food again.

When you feel your new habit has become part of your lifestyle, do another 5-day food journal and pick something else to work on to make more improvements in your eating habits and choices.

7

The Wrap-Up

I've gone over a lot of material in the last 6 chapters.

Have some chapters resonated with you more than others?

Those chapters are probably where you need to start your own new journey to improved health. Go back and re-read those chapters and write out your action plan. Head to the appendix and use the materials there to gain focus and direction.

Some of the changes I'm suggesting you make are not going to be easy. But remember, you don't have to be perfect. You just need to work on getting a little better. Keep in mind some things that take hard work to attain are the most rewarding.

As you work on creating a healthier you, my best advice to you is to stay as consistent as possible. More than anything else, I think consistency wins the game. Just keep plugging along. If you give up— where will that leave you? Certainly worse off than getting a little better every day.

This "life after 40" thing is not always glamorous. I get it. I'm living it right alongside you. Sometimes things hurt. Some days we don't quite move the way we used to. Yet I honestly believe with all my heart that this aging thing is going to be a lot easier on those of us who continue to move, continue to eat well (most of the time) and continue to stay strong. Yes, it will take some effort, but the payoff is priceless.

I wish you fun, smiles and laughter along your new journey to better health and fitness.

If I can be of help to you in any way, please reach out to me at becky@lifeSportFitness.net.

I am committed to your success and I hope that now YOU are, too!

Appendix A

Finding Your Why

Take time and some serious thought to answer the following questions. Write down your responses here and refer back to this page when you begin to get off track with your efforts toward creating healthier habits.

•Why do you desire to be leaner, stronger and healthier?

•Who else is interested in seeing you succeed?

•How will your life be different when you become leaner and more fit?

•What things you will do as a slimmer, more physically fit person that you don't do now?

•What will happen if you DO NOT reach your goals? What will your life be like?

•How will being leaner and more fit impact the people you care about?

• If you get off track and stop your efforts to be healthier and stay at your current weight and fitness level, how will this impact your life and day-to-day activities?

•On a scale from 1-10, how important is it to you that you achieve your goals?

Goals Worksheet

(Remember: Specific, Measurable, Attainable, Realistic, Time-Sensitive)

I will achieve the following in _____weeks:

I will do the following to achieve my goals:

The benefits I will enjoy by reaching my goals include:

Achieving these goals is important to me because:

The obstacles I may encounter as I change my lifestyle include:

I can deal with and overcome these obstacles by:

Appendix B

Workout Ideas

A proper warm up is crucial!

Always, always, always warm up for at least 5-10 minutes before doing any sort of workout. If you're a runner, walking or jogging beforehand is fine. If you're a cyclist, some slow, easy cycling can be your warm up. For things like a strength workout or HIIT workouts, I like my clients to do an "all over" dynamic warm up that prepares their muscles and joints for movement.

Here's simple warm up procedure:

20 heel raises in place (both feet at the same time)
20 toe raises in place (one foot at a time)
20 knee lifts in place

Side step 10 paces left, side step 10 paces back

20 heels to rear end ("butt kickers")

20 half circles with your knees (10 each side)

20 mini squats

10 arm swings overhead

10 arm swings behind your back

10 wall push ups

Easy jog in place for 1 minute

☐

Simple HIIT ideas

The goal with HIIT workouts is to exercise HARD for brief periods and then recover with light exercise for another brief period. You can do this on exercise machines at your health club, or in your own garage or backyard.

Here are two HIIT ideas for your gym:

After a 5 to 10-minute warm up on a stationary bike, treadmill, rower or elliptical:

1) 30 seconds HARD work (about an 8 on a scale of 1-10)

90 seconds recovery (about a 2 or 3 on a scale of 1-10)

This 30:90 segment is ONE round.

Complete 5-10 rounds.

Cool down

2) 60 seconds HARD work (about an 8 on a scale of 1-10)

120 seconds recovery (about a 2 or 3 on a scale of 1-10)

This 30:90 segment is ONE round.

Complete 5-10 rounds.

Cool down

Here are some ideas for your garage or backyard:

After a 5 to 10-minute warm up...

Choose callisthenic-type exercises that get your heart rate up but don't irritate any injuries or sore joints you have.

Examples: Jumping jacks, fast squats, fast lunges, fast jog in place, "Speed skaters", mountain climbers, fast lateral shuffles, med ball slams. If you don't know these terms, just look them up on the web and you're sure to find a picture or video.

I like to pair a couple exercises together so that I mix up the movements and have more variety.

I might choose to do 8 rounds of 40 sec/20 sec time frame and do mountain climbers and speed squats.

Another day I might do a 20 sec/10 sec time frame and choose a fast jog in place and speed skaters.

The combinations of exercises and work/rest ratios are endless. Have some fun with it!

Sample Strength Workouts

I like to create time-efficient strength training programs for busy people using "supersets." In a superset, you pair two non-competing exercises together and complete them one after the other with little to no rest. Sometimes I'll choose one lower body exercise and pair it with an upper body exercise to create a superset. While the lower body exercise is performed, the upper body gets to rest. When the upper body exercise is performed, the lower body is getting some rest. Sometimes I'll create a superset with one pushing exercise and pair it with a pulling exercise.

Using supersets is a fast way to get lots of work done in a short amount of time.

For these workouts, you'll need some exercise tubing with handles and a door attachment.

Workout A

[see Reference section at the end of this book for sample videos with instructions]

Perform exercises in each superset back to back with little to no rest. Perform 1 set of 12-15 reps of the first exercise, then one set of 12-15 reps of the second exercise, then repeat for the number of sets indicated (example: A1, A2, A1, A2, A1, A2, rest, B1, B2, etc.).

Perform 2-3 rounds of each superset.

    A1: Body weight squats
    A2: Wall push up

    B1: Horizontal band row
    B2: Forward step ups on low bench or step

    C1: Squat to curl with band secured low in a door
    C2: Triceps press down with band secured high in door

    D1: Plank (hold for max time)
    D2: The bridge (hold for up to 60 seconds)

Workout B

A1: Lat pull down with band secured high in door

A2: Body weight split squat

B1: Band squat with side leg press out

B2: Dips off bench

C1: Alternating band chest press (band anchored in door above your shoulder height)

C2: Band shoulder press

D1: Side plank (on knee or toes, depending on your strength level) Hold for 30 seconds each side

D2: Bird dog (hold each side for 30 seconds)

☐

About the Author

Becky is not your typical fitness professional. Armed with a graduate degree in kinesiology/physical education, and over 30 years experience in corporate fitness, personal training and scientific research, she is uniquely qualified to provide health and fitness instruction on multiple levels.

In addition to her core competencies in fitness program design, functional exercise, nutrition coaching and working with the "over 40" population, Becky is also a polished public speaker and an excellent contact for the media. She is articulate and credible, and also brings a sense of fun to her presentations and commentary... She is the "kick in the pants" many people need to push themselves to new levels of performance.

Becky began her career in the fitness industry as an intern in a corporate fitness facility in Menlo Park, California. When she completed the internship, Becky was offered a full-time job at the facility, where she stayed throughout graduate school.

Interested in testing her clinical abilities further, she accepted a position as a research exercise physiologist at NASA Ames Research Center after graduate school. During her 10-year tenure at NASA Ames, Becky coordinated a research team tasked with advancing the understanding of the metabolic cost of activity in space. She created a unique set of exercise trials to simulate astronaut extravehicular activity, built a working human performance lab, and published multiple papers on her research findings.

Longing to get back to the "fitness" side of exercise science, Becky created "Exclusively Fit," a health and fitness consulting company, with the goal of seeing a couple of personal training clients per week and pursuing small corporate contracts while still working for NASA. The business eventually outgrew the original goal, and she left NASA to put all her efforts into the business and her passion for health and fitness.

Over the years, she added new services and in 2006 changed the company name to lifeSport Fitness to better reflect the company mission. lifeSport Fitness provides boot camp workouts in and around the San Jose community, and personal training at her fun and inviting private studio in San Jose. Although Becky works with all ages, she specializes in helping busy Silicon Valley residents over the age of 40 feel better, look better and move better with specialized programming designed to help them feel younger longer.

Becky's philosophy of a "fitness lifestyle" is evident in the programs and products she createsfor lifeSport Fitness. She and her team seek to understand each client's goals and design creative ways in which to engage the client in taking an active part in achieving the goal. "It's not just a workout, it's a lifestyle!" she can often be heard saying.

Testimonials highlight Becky's professionalism, quick wit, and her obvious passion and commitment to her clients' success as reasons for choosing lifeSport Fitness. Whether she's coaching a community boot camp for local residents, designing a post-rehab program for a client with a hip replacement, or presenting a motivational lecture at a corporate site, Becky's passion and ability to motivate those around her leaves her clients excited and ready to take action.

In addition to her Master's Degree, Becky is certified as a Health/Fitness Instructor and an Advanced Personal Trainer through the American College of Sports Medicine, and is a certified Personal Fitness Trainer through the American Council on Exercise. She also holds a certification from the American Academy of Health and Fitness Professionals as a Post-Rehab Specialist.

A San Jose native, Becky has been married for 31 years and raised two children with her husband, Matt. When she's not working, Becky can often be found reading or cooking, walking her Golden Retriever or working out at the gym. She has successfully juggled her roles as businesswoman, wife and mother for many years...and as a lover of adventure travel, has also found time to bungee jump in New Zealand, zip line through the jungle canopy in Belize, swim with the dolphins in Mexico and surf in Hawaii.

Testimonials

"I absolutely adore working with Becky. She is so very caring and authentically concerned for my well-being. I have had knee surgeries on both knees over the past few years, and she has helped me gain my strength back and beyond - I haven't felt this good in a very long time. Becky is so passionate about fitness, and she personalizes each session based on my input. I value so much the depth of knowledge she brings about the body and nutrition. I can feel my body positively responding to the workouts, and I just couldn't be more pleased." -DeAnna P. Executive Director of a Non-Profit Organization

"Becky Williamson is flat out THE BOMB! I have been attending personal training sessions with her for about three years now. You won't find a more dedicated, hard-working, and conscientious personal trainer than Becky. Every four weeks or so, she develops a new fitness plan for you so that you're always working towards new fitness goals. She also helps with meal planning and implementing lifestyle changes, if you want to lose weight. Most importantly, you won't find a personal trainer who cares more about you as a human being than Becky." -Melissa S., Technical Writer

"Lost 2 pant sizes in 3 months. Yup, no body cleanses, special foods or drinks; solely going to Becky 2/week for semi-private personal training sessions. Becky PERSONALIZED my work out routine for MY GOALS, and my body issues/limitations. Becky has her Master's Degree and tons of experience in designing programs that will help you succeed. I'm no youngster (considered a "senior" in some circles) so losing 2 pant sizes and getting off blood pressure medications is a big deal for me. Thank you Becky; could NOT have done this without you!" -Carol M. Director of Operations for a Silicon Valley High Tech Firm

"Becky became my personal trainer several years ago when my husband was ill with cancer. I knew I needed to find some stress relief and I also wanted to lose some weight and so it was my lucky day when I found Becky. Those are the reasons I started with Becky, but I've remained with Becky all these years because she is instrumental in keeping me strong and fit. She creates workouts for me that are tailored to my specific needs. She has taught me the value of consistency and she takes me through my workouts with an eye towards building my strength and endurance while at the same time guarding against injury or overuse. I'm 66 and I truly believe I'm stronger today than I was at 36! I owe that to Becky and her ability and expertise." -Kathy W., Retired/Community Volunteer

"Becky provides me with all the tools I need to improve my health and fitness--customized training programs designed

to challenge and strengthen my entire body, expert training and advice to keep me safe and maximize the benefits of my workouts, and a true dedication to help me reach my health and fitness goals." -Linda F., Retired

"I have been a proud member of Becky Williamson's lifeSport Fitness program for years and here is my journey: I was overweight and out of shape when I joined Coach Becky's Fit and Fab Over 40 FitCamp for women one summer. I definitely began feeling stronger and had less pain, but Coach Becky's mantra of "you can't out train a poor diet" is correct. I noticed that when I participated in one of Becky's clean eating challenges, I felt better than ever! Unfortunately, I needed major surgery due to chronic appendicitis, so I stopped working out and stopped eating healthy foods for a while. My arthritis joint pain increased, my hot flashes increased, my weight reached a number I had never seen and my self-esteem plummeted as a result. Early this year, I made a conscious decision to change my diet and get back to regular exercise once and for all. I have been eating real, whole foods since January and participating in Becky's semi-private personal training program. I no longer suffer from arthritis joint pain and hot flashes! Becky carefully plans my workouts in conjunction with my Chiropractor so that I can strengthen my core and build my muscles to support my spine. Becky connects you with other health professionals that can assist you in your fitness journey and she helps you realize that when you are over 40 your health and fitness needs are different and that it is

imperative to recognize this and meet those needs. I am 57 years old and feel amazing once again thanks in large part to Coach Becky and lifeSport Fitness! My kindergarten students have noticed the change in me throughout this school year! My goal is to join the lifeSport Fitness family in the Gladiator Rock and Run mud race later this year. This 57 year older has dropped weight and inches, but more importantly I dropped negative habits and replaced them with positive lifestyle changes. I am grateful! Truly "life is more fun when you're fit." --Lynda E. Kindergarten teacher

"Becky is as real as one can get! She is a dedicated and passionate fitness professional who really cares for her clients' well-being, and works with them individually in attaining their fitness goals. If you are looking to elevate your current fitness/well-being and/or embark on a new regime, look no further. Consider yourself fortunate to have found this special fitness company, lifeSport Fitness, now and not later. Back in the 80's, I was a fitness professional for nearly a decade and have seen a lot of professionals come and go, or lose their passion--not so for Becky. Her workouts are varied, challenging, well thought out and FUN! Becky offers various modifications depending on one's fitness levels and/or physical limitations. For me, I have both a bad back and rheumatoid arthritis, and have been able to keep up over the past three months-with adjustments. In this short amount of time, I have seen a tremendous improvement having lost inches and pounds while decreasing body fat percentage and increasing stamina. Cross training is the quickest and most

effective way to improve fitness in the shortest amount of time. I highly recommend Becky and lifeSport Fitness." - Janine A., Interior Designer

"My experience with Life Sport Fitness has been fantastic! Becky is an incredible coach who supports and pushes you equally well. The workouts are varied and fun. The community is warm and welcoming. Becky has done a great job modifying the workouts for me with my lower back issues and plantar fasciitis. She checks in on my progress regularly, helped me with goal setting, and I've lost 20 pounds!" -Jen W., Stay at home mom

References

Video Links:

Workout A

https://youtu.be/ezKXaqGgDDU

Workout B

https://youtu.be/dg4UpDATkwE

Foam rolling series

Shoulders and chest:

https://www.youtube.com/watch?v=q9uMVMKHmeY

Thighs:
https://youtu.be/HKFAJsQP79E

Hips, butt and hamstrings:
https://youtu.be/bWjAoeUPmxA

Mobility series

Upper Body Mobility:
https://youtu.be/86FC47yBUbg

Lower Body Mobility:
https://youtu.be/gwlhLt2U4kw

29137555R00089

Made in the USA
San Bernardino, CA
12 March 2019